Easy Daily Activities To Boost Seniors' Confidence And Balance

5-Minute Core Workouts With Expert Advice And Step-By-Step Guides

Maritza Mitchell

Table of Contents

CHAPTER ONE

Introduction

Kegel exercises, also known as pelvic floor exercises, are a set of exercises designed to strengthen the pelvic floor muscles. Named after Dr. Arnold Kegel, who first introduced them in the 1940s, these exercises have gained significant recognition for their numerous health benefits.

The pelvic floor is a group of muscles located at the base of the pelvis that support the bladder, uterus, and rectum. These muscles play a crucial role in controlling urinary and bowel function, as well as sexual function. However, factors such as pregnancy, childbirth, aging, obesity, and certain medical conditions can weaken the pelvic floor muscles, leading to issues like urinary incontinence, pelvic organ prolapse, and decreased sexual satisfaction.

Kegel exercises are designed to target and strengthen these muscles, helping to improve their tone and function. The exercises involve contracting and relaxing the pelvic floor muscles in a series of repetitions. The great thing about Kegel exercises is that they can be performed discreetly, as they involve no outward movement and can be done anywhere, anytime.

The benefits of Kegel exercises are manifold. For women, they can help prevent or reduce urinary incontinence, especially after childbirth or during menopause. They can also aid in the recovery of pelvic floor muscles after pregnancy and delivery. Additionally, Kegel exercises can enhance sexual satisfaction by increasing the strength of the pelvic floor muscles, leading to improved orgasms.

Men can also benefit from Kegel exercises. These exercises can help with urinary incontinence, especially after prostate surgery. They may also aid in the treatment of erectile dysfunction by improving blood flow to the genital area and increasing pelvic floor muscle control.

Furthermore, Kegel exercises are relatively simple to learn and can be practiced by individuals of all ages and fitness levels. Regular practice is key to experiencing the full benefits, as it takes time to strengthen the pelvic floor muscles.

Kegel exercises offer numerous advantages for both men and women. By targeting and strengthening the pelvic floor muscles, these exercises can improve urinary and bowel control, prevent pelvic organ prolapse, enhance sexual satisfaction, and contribute to overall well-being. Incorporating Kegel exercises into a daily routine can be a proactive step towards maintaining pelvic floor health and enjoying a higher quality of life.

The Benefits of a Strong Pelvic Floor

A strong pelvic floor provides numerous benefits for both men and women. Some of the advantages:

Improved Bladder Control: Strengthening the pelvic floor muscles can help prevent or reduce urinary incontinence. By enhancing muscle tone and control, individuals can better manage bladder leakage and have improved control over their urinary function.

Enhanced Bowel Function: A strong pelvic floor also plays a role in maintaining bowel control. Weak pelvic floor muscles can contribute to issues such as fecal incontinence and difficulty with bowel movements. Strengthening these muscles can help improve bowel function and reduce the likelihood of these problems.

Prevention of Pelvic Organ Prolapse: Pelvic organ prolapse occurs when the pelvic organs (such as the uterus, bladder, or rectum) descend or bulge into the vaginal area due to weakened pelvic floor muscles. Regular Kegel exercises can help strengthen these muscles and provide support to the pelvic organs, reducing the risk of prolapse.

Improved Sexual Function: Both men and women can benefit from a strong pelvic floor when it comes to sexual satisfaction. Strong muscles in the pelvic floor can lead to increased sensitivity, stronger orgasms, and better control over sexual function. For men, it can also contribute to improved erectile function.

Support During Pregnancy and Postpartum Recovery: Pregnancy and childbirth can place significant strain on the pelvic floor muscles. Strengthening these muscles before and during pregnancy can help support the growing baby, reduce the risk of urinary incontinence during pregnancy, and aid in postpartum recovery by promoting healing and restoring muscle tone.

Prevention of Lower Back Pain: The pelvic floor muscles work in conjunction with the deep abdominal and back muscles to provide stability to the core. A strong pelvic floor can contribute to better posture, reduced strain on the lower back, and decreased risk of lower back pain.

How Kegels Can Improve Your Well-being

Engaging in regular Kegel exercises can have a positive impact on your overall well-being. Here's how:

Convenience and Accessibility: Kegel exercises can be done discreetly and require no special equipment, making them easily accessible to everyone. You can perform them at any time and in any place, whether you're at home, at work, or even while traveling.

Increased Self-awareness: Practicing Kegel exercises involves focusing on the pelvic floor muscles, which increases your awareness of this important area of your body. This heightened body awareness can extend beyond the exercise itself and lead to a better understanding of your overall physical well-being.

Empowerment and Control: Strengthening your pelvic floor muscles gives you a sense of empowerment and control over your body. Knowing that you are actively working to improve your bladder control, sexual function, and overall pelvic health can boost your confidence and well-being.

Preventative Measure: Regularly performing Kegel exercises can act as a preventative measure against pelvic floor disorders. By strengthening these muscles before problems arise, you can reduce the likelihood of experiencing issues such as urinary incontinence, pelvic organ prolapse, or sexual dysfunction later in life.

Improved Quality of Life: A strong and healthy pelvic floor contributes to an improved quality of life. You'll experience fewer limitations or concerns related to bladder and bowel control, enjoy better sexual satisfaction, and have increased confidence in your

body's abilities.

CHAPTER TWO

Anatomy of the Pelvic Floor

To understand the importance of Kegel exercises, it's essential to have a basic understanding of the anatomy of the pelvic floor. The pelvic floor refers to a group of muscles that stretch like a hammock from the pubic bone to the tailbone, forming the bottom of the pelvic cavity. These muscles include:

Pubococcygeus (PC) Muscle: The PC muscle is the most well-known muscle of the pelvic floor. It stretches from the pubic bone to the tailbone and forms a figure-eight shape around the vagina and rectum in women and around the penis and rectum in men.

LevatorAni Muscles: The levatorani muscles consist of three parts: the pubococcygeus, iliococcygeus, and puborectalis. They provide support to the pelvic organs and help maintain continence.

Coccygeus Muscle: The coccygeus muscle, also known as the ischiococcygeus muscle, attaches to the tailbone and supports the pelvic organs.

These muscles work together to support the pelvic organs, maintain continence, and facilitate sexual function. Engaging in Kegel exercises helps strengthen and tone these muscles, leading to improved pelvic floor health and overall well-being.

The Muscles and Structures Involved

To have a deeper understanding of the pelvic floor and its role in supporting various functions, it's helpful to explore the muscles and structures involved. The pelvic floor consists of several layers of muscles, connective tissues, and ligaments that work together to provide support and maintain the integrity of the pelvic region.

LevatorAni Muscles: The levatorani muscles are a group of muscles that form the main component of the pelvic floor. They include the pubococcygeus, iliococcygeus, and puborectalismuscles. These muscles span from the pubic bone to the tailbone and form a sling-like structure that supports the pelvic organs, such as the bladder, uterus, and rectum.

Coccygeus Muscle: The coccygeus muscle, also known as the ischiococcygeus muscle, is located at the back of the pelvic floor. It attaches to the tailbone (coccyx) and helps provide support to the pelvic organs.

Connective Tissues and Ligaments: The pelvic floor is reinforced by various connective tissues and ligaments that help maintain its structural integrity. These include the arcustendineus fasciae pelvis, which supports the front portion of the pelvic floor, and the perineal body, a dense fibrous structure located between the vagina and anus in women (or between the scrotum and anus in men).

The Role of the Pelvic Floor in Support and Function

The pelvic floor plays a crucial role in supporting and maintaining the proper function of several bodily systems. Here are some key functions of the pelvic floor:

Support of Pelvic Organs: One of the primary roles of the pelvic floor is to provide support to the pelvic organs, including the bladder, uterus, and rectum. The muscles and connective tissues of the pelvic floor help keep these organs in their proper position and prevent them from descending or prolapsing.

Urinary Continence: The pelvic floor muscles contribute to urinary continence by actively contracting to close off the urethra and prevent urine leakage. Weak pelvic floor muscles can lead to stress urinary incontinence, where activities such as coughing, sneezing, or lifting can cause involuntary urine leakage.

Bowel Function: The pelvic floor muscles play a role in maintaining bowel control by helping to regulate the opening and closing of the anal sphincter. They assist in the elimination process and prevent fecal incontinence.

Sexual Function: The pelvic floor muscles are involved in sexual function for both men and women. In women, these muscles support the vagina, contribute to vaginal tone, and play a role in orgasmic contractions. In men, the pelvic floor muscles are involved in erectile function and ejaculation.

Preparing for Kegel Exercises

Before starting Kegel exercises, it's important to take a few initial steps to prepare yourself:

Identify the Pelvic Floor Muscles: To effectively perform Kegel exercises, it's essential to correctly identify and engage the pelvic floor muscles. You can begin by trying to stop the flow of urine midstream during urination. The muscles used to do this are the same ones you'll be targeting during Kegel exercises. However, it's important not to make a habit of interrupting the urine flow regularly, as it can lead to incomplete emptying of the bladder.

Find a Comfortable Position: You can perform Kegel exercises in various positions, such as lying down, sitting, or standing. Choose a position that allows you to relax your body and focus on isolating the pelvic floor muscles without unnecessary tension.

Start with Emptying Your Bladder: Before beginning your Kegel exercises, empty your bladder to ensure comfort and avoid any distractions or discomfort during the exercise session.

Gradually Increase Intensity: When starting Kegel exercises, it's recommended to begin with gentle contractions and gradually increase the intensity over time. Start by contracting the pelvic floor muscles for a few seconds and then releasing them. As you become more comfortable and gain strength, you can increase the duration of each contraction and the number of repetitions.

CHAPTER THREE

Assessing Your Pelvic Floor Strength

Before diving into Kegel exercises, it can be helpful to assess your current pelvic floor strength. This assessment will give you a baseline understanding of your muscle tone and help you track your progress over time. Here's a simple method to assess your pelvic floor strength:

Lie down on your back in a comfortable position with your knees bent and feet flat on the floor.

Begin by relaxing your body and taking a few deep breaths to release any tension.

Visualize and focus on your pelvic floor muscles. Imagine the area between your tailbone, pubic bone, and sit bones.

Now, attempt to contract your pelvic floor muscles as if you were trying to lift them upward. Imagine pulling them in and upward.

Pay attention to the sensation and strength of the contraction. Try to hold the contraction for a few seconds and then release.

Assess the strength of your contraction on a scale from 1 to 10, with 1 being very weak and 10 being a strong contraction. Take note of the number to gauge your initial pelvic floor strength.

Identifying Proper Technique and Form

Proper technique and form are crucial for effective Kegel exercises. Follow these guidelines to ensure you are performing them correctly:

Start in a comfortable position, such as sitting or lying down, with your muscles relaxed.

Identify the correct muscles by focusing on the area between your tailbone, pubic bone, and sit bones. It should feel like a subtle lift and squeeze inward.

Avoid tensing your abdominal or buttock muscles. The contraction should be isolated to the pelvic floor.

Breathe naturally throughout the exercise. Avoid holding your breath.

Gradually increase the intensity of the contractions. Start with gentle contractions and progress to stronger, longer contractions as your muscles become stronger.

Aim for a balance between the quality and quantity of contractions. Focus on maintaining a good muscle contraction rather than performing a high number of repetitions.

Basic Kegel Exercises

Now that you've assessed your pelvic floor strength and understand the proper technique, you can start incorporating basic Kegel exercises into your routine. Here's a step-by-step guide:

Begin by relaxing your body and finding a comfortable position.

Contract your pelvic floor muscles by squeezing and lifting them upward. Hold the contraction for a few seconds (aim for 3-5 seconds initially) without holding your breath.

Release the contraction and allow your muscles to relax completely.

Repeat the contraction and relaxation sequence for a set number of repetitions. Start with 5-10 repetitions and gradually increase over time.

Aim to perform Kegel exercises at least three times a day, incorporating them into your daily routine.

As your muscles become stronger, gradually increase the duration of each contraction. Work toward holding each contraction for 10 seconds or more.

Step-by-Step Instructions for Beginners

For beginners, here is a step-by-step guide to performing Kegel exercises:

Find a comfortable position: Start by finding a comfortable position, such as sitting or lying down. Ensure that your body is relaxed, and there is no unnecessary tension in your muscles.

Identify the pelvic floor muscles: Visualize the muscles you will be targeting. Imagine the area between your tailbone, pubic bone, and sit bones. These are the pelvic floor muscles you will engage during the exercises.

Engage the pelvic floor muscles: Squeeze and lift your pelvic floor muscles, as if you are trying to prevent the flow of urine or stop passing gas. Focus on the contraction and avoid tensing other muscles, such as your abdomen or buttocks.

Hold the contraction: Hold the squeeze for a few seconds, aiming for 3-5 seconds initially. Remember to continue breathing naturally during the hold and avoid holding your breath.

Relax the muscles: Release the contraction and allow your pelvic floor muscles to fully relax. Take a moment to rest before proceeding to the next repetition.

Repeat the exercise: Repeat the contraction and relaxation sequence for a set number of repetitions. Start with 5-10 repetitions and gradually increase over time as your muscles become stronger.

Maintain consistency: Aim to perform Kegel exercises at least three times a day, incorporating them into your daily routine. Consistency is important for achieving optimal results.

CHAPTER FOUR

Focusing on Muscle Engagement and Relaxation

During Kegel exercises, it's essential to focus on both muscle engagement and relaxation. Here are some tips to help you maintain the right balance:

Concentrate on muscle engagement: Focus on contracting and squeezing your pelvic floor muscles with the right intensity. You should feel a lift and tightening sensation in the pelvic area.

Avoid overexertion: While it's important to engage the muscles with enough strength, avoid excessive straining or overexertion. The contraction should feel controlled and comfortable, not forced or painful.

Practice proper relaxation: After each contraction, take a moment to fully relax your pelvic floor muscles. Allow them to release any tension and return to their resting state. Relaxation is just as important as muscle engagement.

Breathe naturally: Remember to breathe naturally throughout the exercise. Avoid holding your breath during the contractions, as it can lead to increased tension in the muscles.

Stay mindful of other muscle groups: Focus solely on engaging and relaxing the pelvic floor muscles. Be aware of any tendency to tighten your abdominal, buttock, or thigh muscles. Keep these areas relaxed during the exercise.

Advanced Kegel Exercises

Once you feel comfortable with the basic Kegel exercises and have developed some strength in your pelvic floor muscles, you can progress to more advanced variations. Here are a few examples:

Long holds: Increase the duration of each contraction by gradually extending the hold time. Work your way up to holding the contraction for 10 seconds or longer.

Quick contractions: Perform rapid, quick contractions of the pelvic floor muscles. Squeeze and release the muscles rapidly, aiming for a higher number of repetitions.

Progressive resistance: Use tools designed for pelvic floor exercises, such as Kegel balls or resistance bands. These tools provide added resistance and challenge for the pelvic floor muscles, enhancing their strength and control.

Functional exercises: Incorporate Kegel exercises into functional movements, such as squats or lunges. Engage your pelvic floor muscles while performing these exercises to further strengthen the pelvic floor and improve overall functional stability.

Progressing Your Kegel Routine for Increased Strength and Control

To continue building strength and control in your pelvic floor muscles, it's important to progress your Kegel routine over time. Here are some ways to advance your exercises:

Increase the intensity: Gradually increase the intensity of your contractions. Squeeze your pelvic floor muscles with more force while maintaining good technique and control. Aim for a stronger contraction without straining or holding your breath.

Extend the duration: Lengthen the duration of each contraction. Instead of holding for a few seconds, work your way up to holding for 10 seconds or more. This helps improve endurance and muscle control.

Add more repetitions: Increase the number of repetitions you perform in each session. Start by adding a few extra repetitions and gradually work your way up to a higher number. Focus on quality contractions rather than rushing through the exercise.

Incorporate resistance: Utilize resistance tools designed for pelvic floor exercises, such as Kegel balls or resistance bands. These tools provide additional resistance, challenging your muscles further and promoting strength and control.

Try different positions: Vary your body positions during Kegel exercises. Instead of always lying down or sitting, experiment with standing or incorporating movements like bridges or planks while engaging your pelvic floor muscles. Different positions can engage the muscles in slightly different ways, enhancing their strength and coordination.

Variations and Challenges

Adding variations and challenges to your Kegel routine can keep your exercises interesting and provide additional benefits. Here are some variations you can try:

Elevator Kegels: Imagine your pelvic floor muscles as an elevator. Begin with a gentle contraction at the first floor, then gradually increase the intensity of the contraction as you move up each floor, reaching maximum contraction at the top floor. Slowly release the contraction in reverse order, lowering down the floors.

Quick pulses: Perform quick, rapid pulses of contractions. Squeeze and release your pelvic floor muscles rapidly, aiming for a higher number of repetitions within a set timeframe. This variation improves muscle responsiveness and quick-twitch muscle fibers.

Sideways Kegels: Instead of squeezing your pelvic floor muscles inward, focus on contracting them from side to side.

Imagine drawing the muscles inward toward the right side, then release and draw them inward toward the left side. This variation helps engage different muscle fibers and promotes overall muscle balance.

Integrated movements: Incorporate pelvic floor contractions into functional movements or exercises. For example, engage your pelvic floor while performing squats, lunges, or abdominal exercises. This integration helps strengthen the muscles in a more dynamic and functional manner.

CHAPTER FIVE

Tailoring Kegels for Specific Needs

Kegel exercises can be tailored to address specific needs or conditions. Here are a few examples:

Pregnancy and postpartum: For pregnant individuals or those in the postpartum period, focus on gentle, controlled contractions to maintain pelvic floor strength and support. Avoid overexertion or excessive straining. Consult with a healthcare provider for specific guidance based on your pregnancy or postpartum journey.

Pelvic organ prolapse: If you have pelvic organ prolapse, work with a pelvic floor physical therapist to develop a tailored exercise program. They can guide you in choosing appropriate exercises and provide techniques for managing your condition effectively.

Urinary incontinence: If you're experiencing urinary incontinence, focus on quick contractions to improve the muscles' ability to react and support urinary control. Gradually progress to longer holds to enhance endurance and bladder control.

Menopause-related changes: During menopause, estrogen levels decline, which can affect the pelvic floor. Kegel exercises can help maintain muscle tone and alleviate symptoms like urinary incontinence or vaginal dryness. Regular practice can also improve sexual function and comfort.

Kegels during Pregnancy and Postpartum Recovery

During pregnancy and postpartum recovery, Kegel exercises can play a vital role in maintaining pelvic floor health and supporting the body through these transformative phases. Here's how Kegels can benefit pregnant individuals and aid in postpartum recovery:

During pregnancy:

Improved bladder control: Kegel exercises can help prevent or reduce urinary incontinence, a common issue during pregnancy due to increased pressure on the bladder.

Support for the growing uterus: Strong pelvic floor muscles provide support to the uterus, helping to alleviate discomfort and potentially reducing the risk of pelvic organ prolapse.

Preparation for childbirth: Strengthening the pelvic floor muscles can aid in pushing during labor and promote better recovery postpartum.

During postpartum recovery:

Promoting healing: Kegel exercises can enhance blood circulation in the pelvic area, promoting healing and recovery after childbirth.

Restoring muscle tone: Pregnancy and childbirth can weaken the pelvic floor muscles. Regular Kegel exercises can help restore their strength and tone.

Managing urinary incontinence: Kegels can aid in the recovery of urinary control, which may be affected postpartum.

Addressing pelvic organ prolapse: Strengthening the pelvic floor muscles can help prevent or manage pelvic organ prolapse, a condition where the pelvic organs descend or bulge into the vaginal area.

Addressing Incontinence and Erectile Dysfunction

Kegel exercises are not limited to women; they can also benefit men, particularly in addressing urinary incontinence and erectile dysfunction. Here's how Kegels can help men:

Urinary incontinence: Kegel exercises can strengthen the pelvic floor muscles that support urinary control. They are particularly helpful for men who experience stress urinary incontinence, which is urine leakage during activities like coughing, sneezing, or exercising.

Erectile dysfunction (ED): Kegel exercises can aid in the management of ED. By strengthening the pelvic floor muscles and improving blood circulation to the genital area, Kegels can contribute to better erectile function.

To perform Kegels for men:

Identify the pelvic floor muscles by imagining stopping the flow of urine midstream or by trying to lift the penis with the muscles.

Contract and lift the pelvic floor muscles, holding the contraction for a few seconds.

Release and relax the muscles.

Repeat the contraction and relaxation sequence for a set number of repetitions, gradually increasing the intensity and duration as the muscles become stronger.

Enhancing Your Kegel Routine

To enhance the effectiveness of your Kegel routine, consider incorporating the following techniques and tools:

Biofeedback: Biofeedback devices can provide real-time feedback on your muscle contractions, helping you ensure proper engagement and monitor your progress. These devices can be used alongside Kegel exercises to enhance your awareness and control of the pelvic floor muscles.

Progressive resistance: Gradually introduce resistance by using Kegel balls or resistance bands specifically designed for pelvic floor exercises. These tools add resistance and challenge to the muscles, promoting increased strength and control.

Integrated exercises: Combine Kegel exercises with other movements or exercises to engage the pelvic floor muscles in functional and dynamic ways. For example, incorporate Kegels while doing squats, lunges, or core exercises to promote overall muscle coordination and stability.

Mindfulness and relaxation techniques: Practice deep breathing, meditation, or relaxation techniques alongside your Kegel exercises. These techniques can help reduce overall muscle tension, promote relaxation, and enhance mind-body connection.

CHAPTER FIVE

Pelvic Floor Biofeedback

Pelvic floor biofeedback is a technique that can help maximize the effectiveness of your Kegel exercises by providing real-time feedback on your muscle contractions. It allows you to visualize and monitor the activity of your pelvic floor muscles, ensuring that you are engaging them correctly. How you can incorporate biofeedback into your routine:

Biofeedback devices: There are various types of biofeedback devices available, including vaginal or anal sensors connected to external monitors or smartphone apps. These devices measure the strength and duration of your pelvic floor muscle contractions and provide visual or auditory cues to guide your exercises.

Correct placement: Follow the manufacturer's instructions to correctly place the biofeedback device. Insert the sensor according to the device's guidelines, ensuring that it is comfortably positioned within the vagina or anus.

Focus on the visual or auditory cues: As you contract your pelvic floor muscles, observe the feedback provided by the device. It may include visual cues like graphs or charts, or auditory cues like tones or beeps. Use these cues to guide your contractions and ensure proper muscle engagement.

Adjust and optimize your contractions: Pay attention to the feedback and try to achieve consistent and controlled contractions. Aim for a gradual increase in the strength and duration of your contractions based on the feedback you receive. Strive for smooth, coordinated muscle activation and relaxation.

Track your progress: Take note of your biofeedback results to track your progress over time. Monitor improvements in muscle strength, endurance, and coordination as you continue with your Kegel exercises.

Using Kegel Balls and Weighted Devices Safely and Effectively

Kegel balls and weighted devices can add resistance to your Kegel exercises, enhancing muscle strength and control. Some tips for using these devices safely and effectively:

Consult with a healthcare professional: Before using Kegel balls or weighted devices, it's advisable to consult with a healthcare professional, such as a pelvic floor physical therapist. They can guide you on proper technique, recommend suitable devices, and provide personalized advice based on your needs.

Choose the right size and weight: Select Kegel balls or weighted devices that are appropriate for your level of strength and comfort. Start with lighter weights and gradually increase as your pelvic floor muscles become stronger.

Clean and sanitize the devices: Prior to and after each use, clean the Kegel balls or weighted devices according to the manufacturer's instructions. Maintain good hygiene to prevent any risk of infection.

Use lubrication if needed: If necessary, apply water-based lubricant to the Kegel balls or weighted devices to ensure comfortable insertion and movement.

Practice proper insertion and removal: Follow the instructions provided with the device for proper insertion and removal. Use gentle, controlled movements and avoid any force or discomfort during the process.

Listen to your body: Pay attention to any discomfort, pain, or excessive strain while using Kegel balls or weighted devices. If you experience any negative symptoms, discontinue use and consult with a healthcare professional.

Maintaining Long-Term Pelvic Floor Health

To maintain long-term pelvic floor health beyond Kegel exercises, consider the following practices:

Healthy lifestyle habits: Maintain a healthy weight, engage in regular physical activity, and eat a balanced diet. These lifestyle factors can positively impact your pelvic floor health.

Proper lifting techniques: When lifting heavy objects, engage your pelvic floor muscles and use proper lifting techniques to minimize strain on your pelvic floor.

Posture awareness: Maintain good posture to support optimal alignment and reduce unnecessary pressure on the pelvic floor. Avoid prolonged sitting or standing in positions that place excessive stress on the area.

Avoid chronic straining: Straining during bowel movements or chronic constipation can strain the pelvic floor. Stay hydrated, consume fiber-rich foods, and establish healthy bowel habits to prevent unnecessary strain.

Pelvic floor physical therapy: Consider working with a pelvic floor physical therapist. They can provide personalized guidance, assess your pelvic floor function, and develop a comprehensive plan to address any specific concerns or conditions.

Regular check-ups: Schedule regular check-ups with your healthcare provider to monitor your pelvic floor health. They can offer guidance, address any concerns, and provide appropriate recommendations for your individual needs.

CHAPTER SIX

Integrating Kegels into Your Daily Routine

Integrating Kegel exercises into your daily routine can help ensure consistency and make them a regular part of your life. Here are some tips to incorporate Kegels into your daily routine:

Set reminders: Use alarms or smartphone apps to remind yourself to perform your Kegel exercises at specific times throughout the day. This can help you establish a routine and ensure you don't forget to do them.

Tie them to daily activities: Associate your Kegel exercises with everyday activities. For example, perform Kegels while brushing your teeth, during commercial breaks while watching TV, or while waiting in line. Linking them to existing habits can make it easier to remember and incorporate them into your routine.

Create a dedicated time: Set aside a specific time each day to focus on your Kegel exercises. It could be in the morning, during lunch breaks, or before bedtime. Consistently dedicating time to your exercises helps form a habit.

Make them a part of your workout routine: Incorporate Kegel exercises into your regular workout routine. For instance, you can perform a set of Kegels before or after cardio exercises, strength training, or yoga sessions.

Be adaptable: Adapt your routine to fit your schedule. If you're busy or traveling, modify the duration or intensity of your Kegels, but aim to maintain consistency.

Combining Kegels with Other Fitness Activities

Combining Kegel exercises with other fitness activities can be an effective way to incorporate them into your overall wellness routine. Here are a few ideas:

Pre-activity warm-up: Before engaging in other fitness activities, perform a set of Kegel exercises to warm up and activate your pelvic floor muscles. This can help improve muscle engagement and overall stability during your workout.

Strength training: Incorporate Kegel exercises into your strength training routine. For example, perform a set of Kegels during rest periods between weightlifting sets or integrate them into exercises that target the lower body, such as squats or lunges.

Yoga and Pilates: Combine Kegel exercises with yoga or Pilates movements that focus on core strength and stability. Engage your pelvic floor muscles during poses or exercises that require core activation, such as plank variations or boat pose.

Cardio workouts: Perform Kegels during low-impact cardio activities, such as walking, jogging, or cycling. Engaging your pelvic floor muscles while doing cardio can enhance overall muscle coordination and stability.

Common Challenges and Troubleshooting

Difficulty identifying the correct muscles: If you're having trouble identifying and engaging your pelvic floor muscles, try using biofeedback devices, working with a pelvic floor physical therapist, or seeking guidance from a healthcare professional. They can provide specific techniques to help you locate and engage the correct muscles.

Lack of progress: If you're not experiencing noticeable progress in your pelvic floor strength or function, consider seeking professional guidance. A pelvic floor physical therapist can assess your technique, provide tailored exercises, and address any underlying issues that may be hindering progress.

Lack of motivation or forgetfulness: It's common to feel unmotivated or forgetful when starting any new routine. Set reminders, find an accountability partner, or use apps to track your progress and keep you motivated. Remind yourself of the long-term benefits and the positive impact that regular Kegel exercises can have on your pelvic floor health.

Struggling with consistency: Consistency is key with Kegel exercises. If you're struggling to stay consistent, try to establish a routine by setting specific times each day for your exercises. Make them a priority and approach them as an essential part of your overall well-being.

Pain or discomfort: If you experience pain or discomfort during or after Kegel exercises, consult with a healthcare professional. They can assess your technique, provide recommendations, and address any underlying issues that may be causing the discomfort.

Overcoming Plateaus and Frustration

Reaching a plateau or feeling frustrated with your progress during Kegel exercises is not uncommon. Here are some tips to help you overcome plateaus and stay motivated:

Reassess your technique: Ensure that you are correctly identifying and engaging your pelvic floor muscles. It's possible that over time, you may have developed incorrect habits or lost focus on proper technique. Consult with a healthcare professional or pelvic floor physical therapist to reassess your technique and make any necessary adjustments.

Gradually increase intensity: Plateaus may indicate that your pelvic floor muscles have adapted to your current routine. Gradually increase the intensity of your contractions, duration of holds, or number of repetitions to challenge your muscles further. Progressing gradually helps prevent overexertion and promotes continued strength gains.

Experiment with variations: Introduce variations to your Kegel routine to stimulate your muscles in different ways. Try different positions, incorporate resistance tools, or experiment with different contraction patterns, such as quick pulses or progressive contractions. Adding variety can break through plateaus and keep your routine engaging.

Set achievable goals: Set realistic and achievable goals to track your progress. Break down larger goals into smaller milestones, allowing you to celebrate accomplishments along the way. Feeling a sense of achievement can help maintain motivation and overcome frustration.

Be patient and consistent: Recognize that progress takes time and consistency. Stay committed to your Kegel routine and be patient with yourself. Consistent practice is key to long-term success.

CHAPTER SEVEN

Dealing with Pain or Discomfort during Kegels

Experiencing pain or discomfort during Kegel exercises is not normal and should be addressed. Here's how to deal with pain or discomfort:

Consult with a healthcare professional: If you're experiencing pain or discomfort during Kegels, it's important to consult with a healthcare professional, such as a pelvic floor physical therapist or urologist. They can assess your situation, identify any underlying issues, and provide personalized recommendations.

Adjust technique and intensity: Modify your technique and adjust the intensity of your contractions to ensure you're not overexerting or straining your pelvic floor muscles. Focus on gentle, controlled contractions and gradually increase intensity as your muscles strengthen.

Consider other factors: Pain or discomfort during Kegels can be influenced by factors such as muscle imbalances, hormonal changes, or underlying conditions. A healthcare professional can help identify any contributing factors and develop an appropriate treatment plan.

Practice relaxation techniques: Incorporate relaxation techniques, such as deep breathing or progressive muscle relaxation, before and after your Kegel exercises. Relaxation can help reduce muscle tension and promote comfort.

Modify or pause exercises if necessary: If pain or discomfort persists, your healthcare professional may recommend modifying or temporarily pausing your

Kegel exercises. They can guide you on alternative exercises or treatments to address your specific situation.

Expert Tips for Kegel Success

Some expert tips to enhance your Kegel success:

Consistency is key: Stay consistent with your Kegel exercises. Aim for regular practice, ideally daily, to maximize the benefits and maintain progress.

Mind-body connection: Cultivate a strong mind-body connection by focusing on the sensations and engagement of your pelvic floor muscles during each contraction. Develop a deep awareness of the muscles you are targeting.

Patience and persistence: Understand that strengthening the pelvic floor takes time and effort. Be patient with your progress and stay persistent in your practice.

Seek professional guidance: If you have specific concerns or conditions, consider seeking guidance from a healthcare professional, such as a pelvic floor physical therapist. They can provide personalized advice, assess your technique, and address any unique needs or challenges you may have.

Listen to your body: Pay attention to your body's signals and adjust your exercises accordingly. If something doesn't feel right or if you experience pain or discomfort, consult with a healthcare professional to address any issues.

Advice from Professionals in Pelvic Health

Professionals in pelvic health, such as pelvic floor physical therapists, urologists, and gynecologists, offer valuable insights and advice for maintaining a strong and healthy pelvic floor. Here are some tips from these professionals:

Seek professional guidance: If you have specific concerns or conditions related to your pelvic floor, consult with a healthcare professional specializing in pelvic health. They can provide personalized assessments, guidance, and treatment options tailored to your needs.

Practice proper technique: Focus on proper technique and form during Kegel exercises. A pelvic floor physical therapist can help ensure you're engaging the correct muscles and provide guidance on technique to maximize the effectiveness of your exercises.

Incorporate functional movements: Engage your pelvic floor muscles during functional movements, such as lifting, bending, or twisting, to promote overall pelvic floor strength and stability. A pelvic floor physical therapist can guide you on incorporating these movements effectively.

Emphasize relaxation: Don't forget the importance of relaxation for your pelvic floor. Balancing muscle engagement with relaxation is crucial for maintaining a healthy pelvic floor. Incorporate relaxation techniques, such as deep breathing and mindfulness, into your routine.

Consider multidisciplinary care: In complex cases or if you're facing challenges with your pelvic floor health, consider a multidisciplinary approach. Collaboration between pelvic floor physical therapists, urologists, gynecologists, and other healthcare professionals can provide comprehensive care and address various aspects of your pelvic health.

CHAPTER EIGHT

Strategies for Motivation and Consistency

Maintaining motivation and consistency with your pelvic floor exercises is essential for long-term success. Here are some strategies to help you stay motivated and consistent:

Set specific goals: Set clear and achievable goals for your pelvic floor exercises. Whether it's improving bladder control, reducing pelvic pain, or enhancing sexual function, having specific goals can keep you focused and motivated.

Track your progress: Keep a record of your progress to see how far you've come. Note improvements in strength, endurance, or symptom management. Tracking your progress can provide a sense of accomplishment and encourage you to continue.

Find an accountability partner: Partner with someone who shares similar goals or enlist the support of a friend or family member to hold you accountable. Share your progress, discuss challenges, and celebrate achievements together.

Create a supportive environment: Surround yourself with a supportive environment that encourages your commitment to pelvic floor health. Communicate your needs to your loved ones and ask for their understanding and support.

Make it enjoyable: Find ways to make your pelvic floor exercises enjoyable. Listen to music, watch a favorite show, or engage in activities you love while performing your exercises. Making it enjoyable can increase motivation and make it feel less like a chore.

Addressing Common Concerns and Queries

When it comes to pelvic floor health and Kegel exercises, it's common to have concerns or questions. Here are a few common concerns and some general guidance:

Incontinence during exercises: If you experience urinary leakage during Kegels or other exercises, consult with a healthcare professional. They can assess the cause and provide appropriate strategies to address it, such as modifying the exercise intensity or incorporating additional techniques.

Pelvic pain during exercises: If you experience pelvic pain or discomfort during exercises, consult with a healthcare professional specializing in pelvic health. They can evaluate the cause and recommend modifications, alternative exercises, or treatments to address the pain.

Postpartum recovery: For postpartum individuals, it's common to have questions about pelvic floor recovery. Seek guidance from healthcare professionals specializing in postpartum care, such as pelvic floor physical therapists or obstetricians, for personalized advice on exercises, symptom management, and overall recovery.

Individual variations: Keep in mind that everyone's pelvic floor is unique. The guidance provided here is general, and individual variations may require personalized assessment and recommendations from healthcare professionals.

The Long-Term Benefits of Kegel Exercises

Engaging in regular Kegel exercises and maintaining pelvic floor wellness can provide numerous long-term benefits. Here are some key advantages:

Improved bladder control: Strong pelvic floor muscles can help prevent or reduce urinary incontinence, promoting better control over your bladder. This benefit is particularly significant for women who have experienced pregnancy, childbirth, or menopause, as these life stages can impact bladder control.

Enhanced sexual function: A strong pelvic floor can contribute to improved sexual function and satisfaction. By increasing blood flow to the genital area and enhancing muscle tone, Kegel exercises can aid in arousal, orgasm, and overall sexual well-being.

Prevention and management of pelvic organ prolapse: Pelvic organ prolapse occurs when the pelvic organs, such as the uterus, bladder, or rectum, descend or bulge into the vaginal area. Strengthening the pelvic floor muscles through Kegel exercises can provide support to the pelvic organs and help prevent or manage this condition.

Faster recovery from childbirth: For individuals who have given birth, maintaining pelvic floor strength through Kegel exercises can aid in postpartum recovery. Strong muscles can help support healing and reduce the risk of complications, such as urinary incontinence or pelvic organ prolapse.

Relief from pelvic pain: Kegel exercises can be beneficial for individuals experiencing pelvic pain or discomfort. Strengthening the pelvic floor muscles can help provide support and stability to the pelvis, potentially alleviating symptoms related to conditions like pelvic floor muscle dysfunction or chronic pelvic pain syndrome.

Support during menopause: Hormonal changes during menopause can affect the pelvic floor, leading to symptoms such as urinary incontinence, vaginal dryness, or pelvic organ prolapse. Regular Kegel exercises can help maintain muscle tone, support bladder control, and improve overall pelvic floor health during this life stage.

Conclusion

Maintaining a strong and healthy pelvic floor is crucial for overall well-being. By incorporating regular Kegel exercises, seeking professional guidance when needed, and addressing concerns or challenges along the way, you can promote optimal pelvic floor health.

THE END

9 798328 894067